Sports Nutrition For Endurance Athletes

The Optimum Plan of Nutrition For Athletes

Mariel Warner

This manual contains
information protected under
International Federal Copyright
laws and Treaties.

Any unauthorized reprint or use
of this material is strictly
prohibited. We actively search
for copyright infringement and
you will be prosecuted.

Table of Contents

Introduction

Sports nutrition is nothing short of essential. What you do not know about the athletes that you see on the television, competing in the Olympics and breaking world records is that they have a plan in place that allows them to succeed.

If you will succeed at your sport, you too need to insure that your nutrition is the top of the line. Do you know what you need to do?

Ask yourself these questions:

- Do you know when to eat before your game is to start?

- Do you know what foods are going to help to ultimately win the game if eaten before you compete in the game?

- Do you truly know how much hydration your body needs to power its way through all that you plan to put your body through?

- Did you know that with proper nutrition, the right plan and consistency, your body can do better, perform harder and be more likely to be successful at what you want it to do?

Dedication Counts

When it comes to sports nutrition, there is no reason to

assume that you know it all. In fact, you should be hungry for learning. Learn about what is out there to help enhance your body's performance. Learn about what you should be doing now so that your time on the floor is perfectly optimized. And, learn how to properly take care of yourself to avoid the risk of injury.

When it comes to these things, dedication is the most essential element. You will learn in this book that it takes a lot of hard work and dedication to be successful at sports nutrition. There are no short cuts worth taking either.

Knowledge is the first key to success. You will learn how sports nutrition affects virtually every aspect of your game and how you can better enhance your game by the foods, exercises and processes that you put your body through.

You should dedicate time to work through these steps and suggestions to better your overall performance. As we mentioned, it takes quite a bit of dedication. Therefore, do not expect to eat the right meal and get results right away.

Your body needs you to provide it with the fuel that it needs to do each and every thing that you want to do. Yet, most sports players do not pay enough attention to their goals in sports nutrition. Many make the mistake of believing that if they just work harder that they can do what needs to be done.

Work Smart By Learning First

As an athlete, you need to look at all aspects of the game. Therefore, it is up to you to insure that your game has all the fuel and power behind it to allow you to succeed quickly and effectively.

To get started, read through our book and learn what you are missing. Then, move to using these elements in your everyday life, by adding them in as you go. You should expect it to be hard work. But, when you implement the changes you find here, you can also expect to find results.

It is recommended that you spend some time at least talking with your doctor to insure that your health is at an optimal level before playing any sport or changing your diet drastically. Additionally, if you are facing any physical challenges or taking medications, insure that it is safe for you to follow these recommendations.

Success can and does happen when you look at all areas of your game including sports nutrition.

Chapter 1: What Is Sports Nutrition?

Today is the day that you begin to enhance your game. As an athlete, you already know that you need to work hard at insuring that your skills on the court, field or track are the best they can be.

You want to insure that your body is doing everything in the correct manner from start to finish.

You may spend hours perfecting your movements. You may work to build your muscle to enhance how well you can throw that ball.

Or, you may spend countless hours pushing your body to just

get past that race line by a fraction of a second better.

All of these things are essential parts to being a successful athlete. There is no doubt about that. But, that is not all that you need to handle either.

Off The Court Work Outs

Besides planning your next routine, your next set of reps and your next game, you should be concentrating on your nutrition. Think about it.

What your body eats is what makes it move.

What you put into your body is the fuel it will use to do the things that you want it to do.

What you do not put into your body can not help you to succeed either.

While it may sound hard to determine what the right products are, it does not have to be.

As an athlete, you need to focus your time on sports nutrition as much as you focus it on your workout.

You should take the time to learn about what your body needs, how it reacts to the foods you put into it and how well it will perform based on the fuels you provide it.

The good news is that sports nutrition can be broken down into a much less difficult thing especially in comparison to the workout that you know that you need.

Aspects Of Sports Nutrition

There are several aspects that you need to consider when it comes to sports nutrition. This is the overview of what we will cover here.

- Hydration: Your body needs fluids first and foremost. It needs the right type of fluids and they need to be provided at the right time. This may be a bit tricky at first, but ultimately, without fluids, your body is completely limited in what it can and will do for you.

- Carbohydrates: No, we are not talking about any type of diet here. In fact, carbohydrates are an

- essential building block for your body's workout.

  You need to know when to eat them, what they will do for you, and how much to consume. Luckily, you will find that information here.

- Proteins: Protein is the building block of our body's muscle. Without the right types of proteins in your body, your body can not successfully build muscle groups to accomplish tasks that you want it to.

  You need to learn what you need, when you need to consume it as well as the right products to provide.

- Fats: Are they good or bad? Do you know? Your body does need fat, no matter what those diets tell you.

  But, you need to know what fat is good fat and your body needs to have them delivered at the right time for them to be useful to you.

Doesn't One Diet Work?

Something that is often misunderstood is the reason why there is not just one diet out there that is used for sports nutrition.

If you need certain amounts of foods, specific foods and at the same time, wouldn't everyone be able to follow the same plan along the way?

The answer to this is no. Each and every one of us has a very different body make up. In that, we need various amounts and specific planning in our food consumption.

Another contributing factor to this is our age. Let's face it. Our needs change as we age and our bodies need us to provide them with foods to compensate for those needs.

Even when you are young and fit your body needs something different as you age.

Additionally, the race that you are matters too. Various cultures need various types of foods,

minerals and vitamins.
Remember, bodies developed
over time in various ways.

Therefore what you need is not
the same as what someone
around the globe (or right next
door!) would need.

Finally, your body's size matters
too. Obviously, the larger you
are, the more calories your body
needs to feed your body's cells.
But, that does not mean that you
can just take on a little bit more
here and there.

Even more so, what you plan to
do with your body will effect
what you plan to consume. Will
you physically exert your entire
body or will you simple exert just
your arms? These are plenty of
differences that lie here too.

It All Sounds Confusing

There is no doubt that sports nutrition is a bit complex, but that is only until you break it down and determine what it is that your body truly needs.

When you take the time necessary to balance out all of these factors through a solid sports nutrition plan, you will ultimately be able to succeed at what you need to do, no matter what it is.

Your Goals:

Your goals will follow these needs specifically:

1. Learn when you need to feed your body those foods.

2. Learn what amounts your body will need to be successful.

3. Develop a plan to help you to succeed at sticking with the goals.

4. Work the plan and find success.

That makes it sound easier, right? Throughout the next chapters, things will get easier, we promise! Soon, you will be well on your way to a successful sports nutrition plan that will provide you body with excellent fuel to give you the winning edge you want.

Chapter 2: Hydration Is Key

Keeping your body hydrated is a
very essential part of the process
of sports nutrition. Your body
needs fuel in the form of fluids.
It is a very essential part of your
well being and life in general.

If you do not have enough water
in your body at any given time,
your body will ultimately suffer.
It is a fact of life that can not be
denied.

As an athlete, not providing
yourself with the necessary
amount of water, or limiting it,
can cause you to have numerous
problems including the risk of
serious health complications.

On top of that, your game will suffer without the right amount of water.

Why Water Matters

Without taking you too far back to science class, think about the serious job that water has in your life and in your body.

- It has to be there to move the vitamins, minerals and other nutrients through your body. It keeps blood moving which carries the fuel that your cells need for energy.

- Additionally, water helps to move out the waste products from your cells. This allows them to keep your cells at an optimal level.

- Finally, your body uses fluids to keep the body at the right temperature, there by protecting your health overall.

Can you live without water? No. When it comes to sports nutrition, it is nothing short of essential. How water helps in sports nutrition is important for you to know and to practice.

When your body burns energy, it produces heat. That heat races through your body.

If you think of your body as a car, if the engine gets too hot, it can not perform as it should. Therefore, you will find a way to keep your engine cool, water is a necessity.

Additionally, your body needs to have these fluids to allow you to carry all the nutrients throughout your body. Since you are working on developing muscles, enhancing your physical characteristics, you realize that your body needs those nutrients to get where they need to go.

For that, they need water to push them through.

Water helps your body to grow, but also helps you to repair cells as you work hard at achieving your goals.

The Importance:

If you lose 2% of your body's fluid, your overall performance will considerably drop.

If you lose 5% of your body's fluid, you can find yourself facing heat exhaustion, which is not good. Now, you are barely moving.

If you lose 10% of your body's fluid, you are at risk for heat stroke and even death through dehydration. In other words, game over.

How Much Is Enough?

Do you think you can just drink a glass of water when you are thirsty? Thirst is actually the first sign of dehydration.

If you get to the point of being thirsty, you have already lost at least one percent of your body's fluids and are already putting your body at risk.

There is not too much, drink more than enough to quench your thirst. Do not stop when you are no longer thirsty either.

It is essential that you are always keeping those fluids moving in your body, pumping energy to your cells so that you can perform.

There are plenty of misconceptions out there about how much water is enough water for you to have in your body.

The fact is that your body should not be restricted during your practice, your warm up or during your game.

Your body needs water consistently throughout.

I'm In Good Shape, I Know What My Body Needs

This is a poor attitude to have. When your body tells you it is in need of fluid, it's too far gone to keep performance up. Instead, your mind needs to think, "I need water soon."

Now, if you are a conditioned athlete, well on your way to success, your body will need additional water than that of someone that is, well, farther behind.

- Your body is burning fuel faster and that means more heat is produced quicker.

- On top of that, it is depleting the energy

faster, so fluid needs to
get there faster.

- Your body is probably
  sweating more too, which
  means even more of a
  need.

Tips For Fluids

Here are some basic things that you need to keep in mind when it comes to water.

- Drink water in smaller amounts, more often. This will help to provide a constant level of fluid. If you attempt to drink water too quickly, you get that heavy feeling in your stomach that you just do not need or want to have.

Remember, small, more often.

- Six to eight ounces ever 15 to 20 minutes during your game or during your work out is ideal. If you feel you need more, then increase this amount slightly until you feel comfortable about it.

- Don't go for ice water. You need water that is at the right temperature too. The right temperature is cool water, about 50 to 40 degrees.

  This will help to get rid of the heat in your body but will not sit heavily in your stomach.

- Cool water is absorbed quickly by the body, putting it right to work for you.

- Weigh yourself before and after your workout or competition. Drink eight ounces of water for every pound you have lost for optimum results in your workout. Make it a habit!

- Don't dehydrate yourself for weight loss benefits. While you will drop a few pounds by restricting what you drink, your overall performance will significantly be reduced if you do this.

  Therefore, you need to insure that you follow good hydration steps even when weighing in is important.

- Skip the caffeine. Caffeine is actually like a diuretic and will increase the amount that you have to urinate. Therefore, you are not hydrating yourself, but putting yourself at risk.

  Drinks like this include any type of sports drink that has caffeine as well as things like soda pop, teas, coffee and even foods with high amounts of caffeine.

- A sure way to tell if you are dehydrated or drinking enough water is to pay attention to your urine. Urine that is dark or only a small amount is a sign of dehydration.

  It should be fairly clear and there should be a good amount of it.

Knowing What To Drink

As you can see, we really have pushed the word water here. That's because water is the best type of fluid for you to consume.

Yet, there are many various sports drinks on the market that claim they too can help you.

When considering whether or not you need to drink sports drinks, you need to consider what your practice has been and what your body needs.

To Drink Water: Most of the times you will only need to drink water. Your body does not need fuel from the fluid you drink.

You should drink water whenever you are enjoying a standard workout or game.

Generally, if your physical activity is that of fewer than 90 minutes at a time, you should only need to drink water.

To Drink Sports Drinks:

Now, if your body will have to go for a longer period of time, or you have to compete quite often (several games in just a short amount of time) then you need to consider sports drinks.

When drinking sports drinks, you want to insure that you find those that contain carbohydrates and electrolytes. Your body will need these in these stressful situations.

The sports drink you choose should have less than eight percent in total solids which includes both carbohydrates as well as electrolytes.

If you go with something that has more, it is not easily absorbed into your body, delaying any benefit it may have. Dilute sports drinks by 50% if they contain over this amount.

Avoid fructose sports drinks. Look at the label. If you see it has fructose as the only source of carbohydrates, then you will want to avoid it. It will take your body longer to use these products and delay results even further.

Juices

You can use juices at the same time that you would use the sports drinks, only during long, hard sessions of endurance.

If you do use these products to help you to gain back some of your body's necessary power, you will want to dilute them. To do this, dilute an equal about of fruit juice to the same amount of water.

You will do this because standard fruit juices have a high concentration of carbohydrates. This amount is far too much for your body to use easily.

You should consider fruit juices such as orange juice to refuel on.

When you use these tips to help you keep your body fueled, you will find yourself completely ready to perform at a high level. It is necessary to insure you provide optimum levels of hydration as it applies to sports nutrition.

Chapter 3: Fueling Your Body

Food. Your body needs this simple tool to help it to do virtually every single thing that it has to do. From breathing to walking to playing your game, your body depends on food to fuel it.

While water is essential to life, food is essential to performance. Without the right amounts, types and timing for the food you eat, your body will not be able to reach its highest level of performance no matter what you plan to do.

There is no workout that will work for your body more so than the fuel that you give it. It has a direct relation to your performance and therefore is one of the building blocks in successful sports nutrition.

The Balanced Win

As an athlete, your specific needs are your own, but there is no doubt that if you want to win at physical activity, you need your body to have a balanced diet. You probably have heard this many number of times, but it is the same as day one.

You need to consume a balanced diet of foods to be successful.

The combination of foods will provide your body with all the essential building blocks that it needs. This includes vitamins, minerals, fats, carbohydrates, and proteins. Each of these elements plays their own role, one that is crucial to your success.

Think of food as a team effort. You know that you are only as good as your team is, right? When you do not provide all of the right nutrients to your body, to limit them, they can not perform as a team and then the overall whole suffers.

How many times does the star athlete go down in a game and the team crumbles around them? Or, how many times does someone that is a smaller asset and the star can not longer hold the team up? The same is true for food.

The body needs each one of these pieces for the whole to work. The goal that you have is to learn what it needs and how it needs them to get the whole working well.

Over the course of the next chapters, you will better learn what each element plays in the whole race. But, for now, we want to take you back to grade school where you learned what your body needs to sustain a good overall healthy lifestyle.

Lucky for you, this same information will apply to your own health in sports nutrition now.

Foods: A Plan For Successful Diet Management

Eating food is a must, of course, but what you eat is just as important as how much you eat. So, let's break it all down for you.

Do you remember the food pyramid from school? That is the ideal thing for you to use for your basic sport nutrition education.

While we will tweak it later, this is the overall best thing to use to determine where your level of nutrition stacks up.

What You Need

Here's the breakdown for you. But, we want to strongly inform you that what is listed here is the minimum of what your body needs to perform. The more you demand from your body, the more it will need. We will go into more detail on what that will include later.

Dairy Group:

Your body needs dairy to provide your body with calcium. Proteins, vitamin A, and riboflavin are also found in dairy, making it necessary for good nutrition.

You should consume at least 3 servings per day which is about 8 ounces of liquid or about one and a half ounces of solids.

You will find dairy in milk, yogurt, and cheese. You should limit the amount of fat that comes in from these items though. Low fat products increase the good while decreasing the bad.

Vegetable Group:

Vegetables are ideal. You will get many of your nutrients like vitamins and minerals from vegetables. You need an all around good variety of foods to fit this need.

To balance what you eat, try to eat lots of different colors and look for dark colors for more benefit.

You should have five servings of vegetables per day which is about half of a cup of raw or cooked vegetables, one cup of leafy vegetables or six ounces of juice.

Great choices in vegetables include tomatoes, broccoli, and Brussels sprouts for their high levels of vitamin C. For vitamin C, go with carrots, sweet potatoes, pumpkin, greens, and spinach.

Darker colors, like dark greens, deep reds, oranges and yellows are ideal for a good overall nutritional value.

Meat Group:

With meat comes protein, the very building block for muscles. Therefore you need to insure that you get enough protein in your diet to allow you to build your strength. Meats also include iron, thiamin, riboflavin, niacin and zinc.

You need to consume three servings per day in meats. This is about three ounces of cooked meats, two eggs, one cup of cooked beans or lentils, or four tablespoons of peanut butter.

Good choices include lean amounts of beef, pork, lamb, poultry, dry peas and beans, peanut butter and eggs.

Grains Group:

You will learn that carbohydrates are a necessary building block for energy in the body and many will come from grains. They provide complex carbohydrates that you need including starch and fiber.

Additionally, they contain protein, the B vitamin group and iron.

You need to consume eleven servings of carbohydrates per day. This is about one slice of bread, three or four crackers, half of a coup of cereal, rice or pasta,

and one ounce of breakfast
cereal.

Good choices for sports nutrition
include grains that are whole
grain. In this group you find
cereals, bread, pasta, and rice.
Whole grains are a must.

Fruits:

Fruits are another source of
many of your necessary minerals
and vitamins. They have vitamin
C which is powerful and can be
found in your citrus foods.

Additionally, melons,
strawberries and blueberries are
all great sources. Apricots are
great for Vitamin A.

You need to consume four
servings per day in fruits which is
one whole fruit item like eating a

banana or an apple. Half of a grapefruit, six ounces of fruit juice, or a quarter of a cup of dried fruits equals a serving.

Calories

When it comes to your fuel intake, you also need to keep in mind that the more that you do, the more that you will need to provide your body in fuel. If you want to go farther in your vehicle, it needs more gas right? The same here is true.

We monitor how much we intake by calorie count. The average person will need to consume about 3000 calories per day. If you are intensely athletic, you should increase this to 5000 calories a day.

But, you must do this in the right manner. That is, you should increase it through eating additions of all food groups that we have mentioned and it should be done with lean foods rather that fatty foods.

Depending on the amount of exercise, practice, competition and physical exertion that you need to put out will ultimately determine the amount of calories you need.

You do not want to eat too many so that you gain weight in fat, but you do want to provide enough for weight gain in muscle as well as for energy use.

Tips To Remember

1. Eat often, but eat less. Your body should not need to wait hours before its next meal. You need to provide it with the fuel it needs consistently. Eat a meal every few hours that is much smaller.

2. Snacks are the ideal meal between big meals. But, do not go for empty calories or poor nutrition. Great choices for snacks are vegetables, fruits, salads, and nuts. These provide high levels of minerals and vitamins your body is craving.

3. Get your energy from all the food groups.

Carbohydrates are ideal for times when you are pushing yourself hard. They are perfect for a workout. But, you do not want to cover them with bad stuff either. Go without the butter and without the dressings.

4. Breakfast is essential. Your body needs a kick start in the morning to get the metabolism moving. It also gets your body working the right way from the start. Don't skip it.

5. Skip late night meals. They will not provide you with anything necessary for your health. You need to provide your body with nutrients so that it can

do things. Food is fuel,
not needed for sleeping!

In The Next Chapters

In the next chapters, we will
break down all the needs that
you have and tell you how to
balance the carbohydrates, the
proteins, the fats and other
elements in your diet.

It is important to know when to
eat and how these elements of
your diet power your diet and
your sports abilities.

Chapter 4: Carbohydrates Role

We hear a lot about carbohydrates today. Often, they are called bad and unhealthy. Yet, this is not true.

Go back to an analogy of the team. As a team, nutrients work together but if you take one away or lessen the amount you eat of it, you drastically lessen the quality of the rest of the team.

In this case, you need to realize that it is necessary for your body to have the carbohydrates that it needs to power through your body's demands. Carbohydrates are nothing short of essential.

As you will learn here and throughout this book, the best thing that you can do is to provide your body with the right type of food. So, while we say carbohydrates are good, that does not mean that any carbohydrate are good.

You should always look for whole grains when it comes to carbohydrates and you should look for things that are not full of sugars, bad fats and processed foods.

Did that just end your food tastes? It shouldn't.

The Role Of Carbs

As part of a balanced diet, carbohydrates are a necessary part, but what do they do to your body when it comes to sports nutrition?

In the world of sports nutrition, carbohydrates play a large role. They are necessary because they provide an essential source of foods for your nutrition. If you look back at your food pyramid, you will notice that you are supposed to consume 11 servings per day of grains.

Grains make up most of your carbohydrate intake, but that is not all. In fact, you will intake carbohydrates when you eat fruits, vegetables and other foods as well. Most commonly, starch foods will contain mostly carbohydrates.

Carbohydrates should be consumed at 65 to 70 percent of your body's calories!

How They Effect Your Body

Carbohydrates are necessary for the production of energy in your body.

- The body will take carbohydrates and convent them to sugars for easy consumption.

- The starch in carbohydrates is used for energy in the form of glucose (the sugar) to power the body through exercises.

- Carbohydrates are also stored in your liver as well as in the muscle tissues throughout your body. This is called glycogen.

- Carbohydrates give you a high power boost of

energy for a short time period.

- When the body does run out of carbohydrates in this type of fuel, it will then burn other elements including fat and then it will go to protein to use for energy output.

- When your body goes to fat usage for energy, the level of performance you get will drop.

- When the body goes from fat to protein, it is beginning to take apart muscle mass which is counteractive and therefore will cause performance to further drop significantly.

- Not enough carbohydrates when you

begin to exercise, play your game, or physically exert yourself and your body will resort to turning to stored fat and stored protein.

- Do not exercise heavily for more than 60 minutes without consuming any carbohydrates.

- Do not do anything high intensity too much without any carbohydrates available to power your body through fuel.

- Keep the amount of events, games, or physical exertions for one day or several days, minimal or, add additional carbohydrates to your diet during this very intense period.

Points To Remember

There are two things that you need to remember when it comes to carbohydrates:

1. Eat quite a few carbohydrate foods for the several days before your event, heavy exercise routine, your exercising routine or any other time in which you will need lots of energy available. This will help to load your muscles with glycogen: fuel for your body's needs.

2. If you will be participating in a high intensity, long term event or several events over a short period of time or other instances where you will

need to burn energy for an extended period of time, replenish your carbohydrates as you go. You can do this with fruit juice or through carbohydrate drinks like the ones we talked about earlier.

Carbohydrate Loading: Good Or Bad For You?

If you are considering carbohydrate loading, which is the method of adding additional carbohydrates to your diet prior to a race, event or competition, you need to look at what your needs are for that event as well as what your physical condition is for it.

The goal of carbohydrate loading, which is also known as glycogen loading, is quite straight forward. Remember how we said that your body takes carbohydrates and breaks them down into glycogen?

Glycogen is then stored in your muscles as well as in your liver. When your body needs to access reserved or stored carbohydrates, it will go to the stored glycogen first before it attempts to break down fats and proteins.

When you are carbohydrate loading, you are packing your liver and muscles full of glycogen to allow your body to have those reserves full and readily accessible to your body when the time does come.

It can be quite helpful to an athlete to have glycogen ready to go, but it should be done effectively and with good sources of carbohydrates.

How To Use Carbohydrate Loading

If you would like to see the benefits of carbohydrate loading, you will want to consider this.

- Several days before you will need to use the stored glycogen for your race or competition, eat a diet that is rich in protein, high in fat and low in carbohydrates.

- This is accompanied by the intense training workouts you are probably doing to get ready and in shape for your competition.

- This will deplete the body's reserves of glycogen, something that needs to be done first.

- Now that it is nearly depleted, two to three days before your event, you will be ready to carbohydrate load your body. Eat a very high amount of carbohydrates during this period of time. This should be foods from the grain group.

- You should not be doing any type of extraneous exercising during this period of time. You do not want the body to burn through those stored glycogen carbohydrates. It also gives your body the ability to repair damage from the last workouts to enable you to work harder on the day of the event.

When it comes to this type of activity, really take the time to learn if you need to use it. You should not need to use carbohydrate loading unless you need your endurance level to remain high for an extended amount of time, such as in a long running race or in a bike race.

You should also realize that you probably will not do well in your high protein phase of this carbohydrate session.

Finally, most athletes will eat an overall high amount of carbohydrates during their exercise regimens as it is the fuel your body needs.

But this routine for carbohydrate loading should only be done as preparation for high intensity, long events, not as a regular routine.

Chapter 5: The Need For Protein

Another aspect of the athlete's sports nutrition is that of protein. Protein is yet another fundamental building block that you need to incorporate into your diet in the right manner in order to succeed at building your body into an energy producing machine so you can win at your game, whatever that is.

Protein is a necessary element in your diet but you should take note that you do not need to go on an all protein diet by any means.

In fact, too much protein can be detrimental to your actual results.

Again, we can bring back that team. Here, without protein or with not enough protein, your body will have a difficult time building up to the endurance level that it needs.

It will not have enough of what it needs to build muscle tissue so that your workouts are meaningful.

As part of your body's necessary team for success, protein intake should be monitored carefully, especially around your events and competitions.

What's Protein?

Protein comes from most products that are in the meat group. It comes from fish, beef, poultry, pork, lamb, eggs, nuts and dairy products as well.

The amount of protein you eat will vary but it should be consumed at about 15 percent of the total amount of calories that you take in, still a significant amount and right behind that of carbohydrates.

While carbohydrates will be used to provide your body with the energy it needs to go from one place to the next, protein is essential for building the body up so that it has the physical capabilities for that to happen.

Proteins are what give your body the necessary abilities to build new tissue in your body, to repair damaged tissues in your body and to maintain fluids throughout your body.

They do other things as well, but for the athlete, this is the most essential aspect to know.

What is important to note about protein is the body's inability to store excess amounts of protein. Unlike that of the carbohydrate, it can not store it up to use when needed.

The body will use protein for its needs and then it will burn it for energy. If it does not need to use it for this matter, then it will convert the protein into fat and pack it onto your thighs, and everywhere else for that matter.

Therefore, balancing the right amount of protein in your diet is essential to the athlete competing to win.

What Do I Need?

When it comes to protein, there are several things that you need to carefully consider. How much you need is varied depending on these characteristics:

- What type of exercising are you doing?

- What level of exercise are you doing in terms of intensity?

- How long will you be performing these exercises for?

- The total calories you are consuming also plays a role in how much you should intake.

- And, this also is dependent on the amount of carbohydrates that you are consuming.

Your level of fitness plays a role in the amount of protein your body needs. If you are physically active, as most athletes are, your body will need more protein than if you were not active or were minimally so.

When you first begin your exercise program, you will need to increase the amount of protein calories you are taking in as well.

That is, you should increase them because your body will be building muscles faster and toning them faster at this time.

Your body will need additional protein calories then, but this will soon taper off when there is less muscle and tissue building taking place.

In your exercise type, your level of protein is very important. This is determined by how intense the exercise you are doing will be as well as the duration of the exercise as well.

Those that need endurance for a longer period of time will in fact need more protein so that it can be used to burn as fuel when you do run out of carbohydrates.

Those that are endurance runners, for example, need to have more protein in their diets than those that are short duration athletes.

If you are a body builder or you will be doing strength building exercises in general, you need to increase the intake of protein that you have as well.

Calorie intake also makes a difference. If you eat the wrong amount of food, generally speaking, your body will resort to burning protein as fuel.

If you do not eat enough calories in your diet, your body has to go to the protein to burn for energy. It burns more protein then so you will need to increase the protein you eat.

Carbohydrates that you take in also play a role in the amount of protein that you need. If you do not eat enough carbohydrates, your body has to use protein to burn for energy.

If you start a race with lower levels of glycogen, you will end up burning more protein than you would otherwise. In fact, you can burn up to 10 percent more this way.

Of course, we said that you want your body to burn carbohydrates as opposed to burning proteins!

The Truth About High Protein

No, we are not talking about the weight loss diets that you will only consume protein for, well, the rest of your life.

Remember our team analogy, that's not a good diet to be on for anyone!

What we are talking about is muscle building high protein

diets. While an athlete that is working to build muscle mass does need to intake more protein calories, it is where you get these from that matter.

You are sure to have seen high protein meals and drinks on the market. These are used to target those that are looking to add additional grams of protein to the diet easily.

In sports nutrition, it is not necessary for you to resort to those products unless you do not eat the right amounts of proteins from the start.

It is commonly believed that eating high protein supplements like these is not necessary as long as you naturally increase the amount of protein calories that you take in.

To do this, add into your diet

more low fat, high protein foods just as a natural addition to your diet. This may include eating more meats like poultry, beef, pork, fish and nuts to your diet.

Also, remember that high protein diets are only geared to those that are looking to build muscle mass.

- If you are just starting out in your exercise routine, you will need additional calories coming from protein.

- If you are looking to build muscle mass, such as with body building, you too will need to increase the amount of protein you intake in a high protein diet.

The standard athlete does not necessarily have to eat more protein than the 15 percent that we mentioned unless they fall under one of these categories.

In addition to this, it is important to note that many high protein diet supplements and foods can do more harm that they are worth.

For example, they are known to cause people to lose their appetite, which in turn causes them not to get the necessary carbohydrates they need for sustained exercise.

Additional problems are dehydration, diarrhea and too much pressure on the kidneys to perform.

Maintaining the amount of protein that you but into your diet is crucial!

Chapter 6: The Story With Fats

You have heard a lot about fats in your life, no doubt. But, when it comes to sports nutrition, none of that really matters.

One thing you need to realize is that when the stakes are higher, as in when your body needs to perform at a higher level, it is important for you to provide it with the foundation to do so.

Many of the things you will read here will not provide a balanced diet outside of sports. These things are geared to provide your body with the foundation of producing higher amounts of energy and therefore endurance.

When it comes to fat, there is much to learn as well.

What Is Fat?

Fat is a product that you ingest when you eat foods. While there is not just one food group that it comes from, there are many things that you need to realize that do contain higher amounts of fat.

Fat comes from anything that is from animals. This type of fat is called saturated fat and is the worst of the two types. This would include:

- Meats of all types have fat; even lean meats will have some levels of fat in them.

- Eggs have a high fat amount in it.

- Milk, even low fat milk, still has a good amount of fat within it.

- Cheese too may be low fat, but will still have a good amount of fat in it.

Unsaturated fats are fats that come from vegetable products. Your oils are high producers of fat. It comes from vegetables of all types, but in different amounts.

Unsaturated fats are a better, healthier version of fat to have within your body.

How Much To Consume

When it comes to how much fat you should be consuming, it is not as complex as that of your carbohydrate or your protein calories.

In fat intake, you should not consume more than 25 to 30 percent of your calories in fat. Generally speaking, this is not hard to do, unless you are used to eating deep fried products or those that are covered with saturated butters and sauces.

Did we again just throw off your daily diet intake? Sorry, but the body needs to be regulated here.

Fat In The Body

Your body does need some fat though. Have you heard of those diets in which people will cut out nearly all the fat in their diet? Yes, you are right.

Look back at our team playing theory.

You need to consume a balanced diet of products, ones that will incorporate various amounts of fats to balance your needs.

Your body does only need a small amount of fat though. It needs this to help with several functions. From a sports nutrition stand point, fat is used to burn as energy. Remember when we said that our bodies will first burn carbohydrates and then will result to proteins?

Fat is next on the list of energy sources when there is not enough carbohydrates or glycogen available to burn.

So, why not load up on the amounts of fat that your body consumes as it seems to be a fundamental part of energy and fuel? There are many reasons.

The main reason that you do not need to eat excess amounts of fat is because of how unhealthy it is to the rest of your body.

Too much fat in your body can cause a number of health problems starting with heart disease, the number one killer in the United States. It can also lead to cancers, complications of other conditions and just an overall unhealthy lifestyle that is anything but beneficial to the body or to your sports life.

If you are consuming too much fat, you are probably not getting the right amount of carbohydrates that you need as well.

Even more so, when we talked about carbohydrates, we told you that carbohydrates are easily burned by the body for energy. When it comes to burning fat, it is harder for the body to do.

Therefore, fat should not be considered as a needed element to consume in order to burn as energy for the body.

Three Times Fats Are Used

There are three main times in which fat will be used to burn energy in your body or will be needed for you to have on hand for that reason.

1. If you are participating in extreme or intense exercise, your body will need more energy to burn then you have stored in glycogen or in carbohydrates readily available. It will then turn to stored fat for help in providing you with the energy that you need.

2. When your body is at rest or you are just doing low to moderate amounts of work, your body will then primarily use fat to burn as fuel. During this time, just small amounts of fat will actually be burned, though.

3. If you continue to exercise for long periods of time, such as when you do during a marathon, a long endurance race of any type, your body then needs to tap into fat stores to help it to power through all of these needs.

When it comes to fat and sports nutrition, it is something that you really do need to monitor. If you should consume quite a bit of fatty foods, especially those that are made from saturated fats, you are putting your health at risk.

As far as sports nutrition goes, too much fat can cause your performance to slip. The body does not perform as well as it does with carbohydrates or even by burning protein when you are consuming fats.

Chapter 7: Meal Planning
For Your Game

We have broken it all down for you now. Think you are done, ready to go out there and win at your game?

Not just yet, but soon you will be. As you have learned, there is much to getting your body fed the right amounts of fuel at the right time. It is not easy, but it can and does get done everyday by athletes.

Now that we have broken it all down, we can start to put it back together for you.

To do that, we will work on developing a pre game plan for what you should eat, how you should eat it and how much you should eat prior to your athletic performance.

What you eat right before your competition or performance is a direct reflection of what will happen in that performance. In short, your body will only perform to the level that you have prepped it for.

Have you ever been mid event only to feel so tired that you just feel as if you can not take just one more step? This is your fuel running out.

If you are a car, you are done, on the side of the road waiting for your driver to refuel you. But, if the driver prepared before the start of the drive, you would not have any problem hitting the destination and doing it in the way that you want to succeed.

It's Starts Before Game Day

One thing to take note of is the fact that your pre game planning needs to start several days before you actually head out there to compete.

Don't plan to just wake up, eat breakfast and hit the run. You need to plan several days in advance for what will happen just this one day, this one race, this one competition.

As we talked about, the goal is to store up enough glycogen in your body so that you can withstand what needs to be done during your event. We are not talking about carbohydrate loading, mind you.

This would be something you only do when you are going for a long intense effort, not for a standard event that is short lived.

By following a good regimen, your body will be better able to meet the needs it will be required to meet. The right plan can also do things that you may not have thought of needing to consider.

1. It can help to keep your blood sugar at a level amount which controls your energy amounts.

2. It helps to build up your muscle and liver glycogen that we have talked about.

3. You will have virtually nothing in your stomach at game time, meaning that you do not have that

full, can't do a thing
feeling.

4. It helps you to avoid
    hunger as well as an
    upset stomach during
    your event.

5. It finally helps to keep
    your body completely
    hydrated so that your
    energy is flowing where it
    needs to be during your
    event.

Now, there are many ways to
take the next plan, but we want
you to know that this is just a
basic plan. It is not necessarily
perfect for everyone and
definitely will not provide you
with a perfect outcome to your
events.

But, it can help you to get back
on track, get your body ready to

go and then allow you to change it up as you see necessarily down the road.

Things You Have To Know

As someone that is competing in an athletic event, you need to position yourself for success and the only way that you can really do that is to provide the necessary fuel for your body.

Here's a break down of what you should be doing now.

- Your last meal before your event should happen no shorter than three full hours before your event. Do not try to eat a meal right before.

Your stomach will be upset, will weigh you down and you will feel no benefit from the foods consumed.

- Keep yourself fully hydrated for several days before your event. Of course, you really do want to try to always remain hydrated but remember that it takes the body time to re-hydrate itself (sometimes days even) when you are dehydrated.

- Now, the meal before your event should be something that is high in starch. It should be carbohydrate full to allow your body to easily digest it, quickly and effectively, so that you have the necessary power to go.

It is also helpful in maintaining your body's blood sugar level as well.

- In that meal and maybe even the one before it, limit the amount of protein that you are consuming. Remember, proteins are not meant to be energy. They are harder for the body to digest and will hold you back ultimately.

You definitely do not want to end up dehydrated because you have consumed too many proteins either.

- Do not eat foods or drink fluids that contain caffeine. As you remember, caffeine is something that can cause your body to dehydrate and simply not give you the right outcome.

Even energy drinks that have caffeine in them will ultimately restrict your abilities in the events.

- Do not eat foods that have not been found in our food chart. You do not want to eat foods that are high in sugar at all.

This will really not do anything but keep your energy waning rather than help you to power through.

- Drop the oils. We also mentioned how fats are

not a good thing for
your body. So,
especially in this last
meal before your event,
limit the foods that you
eat that are high in fats.

Do not forget to consider
the butter on your
pancakes and the oil in
your salad dressings. You
will find fats everywhere
and they need to be
noticed.

What Should I Eat?

So you know what you want to
eat on that last meal, right? You
are right, it does seem limiting,
but really, it does not have to be.

Go back to our breakdown of
foods that fit well within the

categories of carbohydrates (check out the grains!) in proteins (meats and dairy products) and avoid those foods that you find are high in fats.

Really, you can eat anything you want as long as it fits within the calorie suggestions and in the food groups we have listed there.

Chapter 8: Foods That Work Well

Okay, so you would like some help in determining what foods are ideal for the pre game meal or maybe just an overall look at what you should be eating.

Here's a break down that will help you.

Foods High In Carbohydrates

The first and most important aspect of sports nutrition is to provide your body with the building blocks of what it needs to perform. That is in the carbohydrates.

Here are some foods that are ideal to consume as high

carbohydrate foods. In other words, these are the foods to eat prior to your game, your competition or your events.

Potatoes

Potatoes are high in starch and carbohydrates. They make for the ideal pre event meal choice. You can eat them any way that you would like including baking them, mashing them, pan frying them, broiling them and so on. Avoid deep frying them (no French fries please!)

Also you need to be careful with what you put on them. Things like butter or gravy can be heavily saturated with fats that you do not need. Sour cream goes along with that.

If you can't live without it, then consider cutting down on how much of the condiment or additional additive you place on them.

Pasta

Even if you are not Italian, you probably have lots of pasta in your home. It's a quick and easy meal and it's great for sports nutrition preparations.

There are many choices out there including a variety of noodle shapes from macaroni to ravioli, to spaghetti and everything in between.

You can top it with spaghetti sauce or go without.

Be careful when you add oils, butter, or heavy sauces to the pasta though. You should also not top it with too much meat either, especially if this is pre game a experience. Cheese too should be avoided or kept at a minimum especially if it contains lots of fat.

Rice

When it comes to rice products, you have all types of options. Consider mixing the rice with vegetables if you would like to. Add some hot peppers for taste, but do not over do it. You do not want to have a stomach ache prior to your event.

Again, you should limit the things that you place into the rice. It should not be things that are high in saturated fats. Avoid gravy, butters or other heavy cream sauces.

Cereals

Most cereals are okay for you to use. But, you need to flip them over and look at what is in them. You want to avoid foods that are high in sugar or fats. Believe it or not, many cereals are.

You should consider foods like oatmeal and other warm cereal type foods, but make sure that you again, check what is in them.

Always top the cereal with low fat milk products. Avoid adding additional sugar to them. Again, this will just provide the wrong power to you.

Bread

Bread is a big yes! There are plenty of products that are ideal here. From slices of breads to rolls, you have many choices to pick from.

But, again, you really do need to limit what you put on the breads. You should not top them with lots of butter or fill them with high protein or high fat foods. Spreads and other products that are added that are high in fat will cause the benefits to be weighed down.

Fruits

A large confusion has to do with fruits. Because they are sweet, they seem to be something that is not good for us. While they do have sugar in them, it is natural sugars that allow our bodies to better stay hydrated and to have the carbohydrates that we need. Therefore, these types of juices

are quite worthwhile to
consume.

Your options are many and
should include things like
oranges, bananas, and apples. In
the form of whole fruits, most
are easy for your body to digest
and will provide the necessary
nutrition that you need.

In the way of juices, you will want
to look at what is in them. You
do not want your fruit juices to
have more than 8 percent of
carbohydrates or electrolytes as
this will make them harder for
your body to digest.

Dairy Products

If you have to have your milk
with your breakfast by all means
have it. Actually, any and all low
fat dairy products are perfect for
the sports nutrition guide. Try a

variety of things including low fat milk, low fat cheeses, low fat yogurts and others.

Again, avoid things that are high in fat or that are added to the dairy products such as chocolate.

Chapter 9: Foods That Will Hurt

Unfortunately, not all foods in the world are good for our sports nutrition diet.

But, remember, giving up food to win the race, the marathon or to find ultimate fitness is a reward far better than any food product out there.

Giving up on these things does not have to be permanent, unless you plan to be athletic all that time. In other words, you do not have to restrict yourself from these foods forever. In fact, you may be able to squeeze something in when you are not performing or practicing, if you dare take a break!

Here are some foods you just should avoid and reasons why they are anything but helpful to your overall performance and expectations.

1. Candy. There we said it. You have to give up candy products because of the amount of sugars in them. They can throw off your blood sugar and cause you to have less than ideal results in your performance.

   They can also make you feel awful after only a few minutes of being in your system. The reason is that they create a natural rush that can only be sustained for a short period of time.

2. Caffeine. We have already mentioned this in

our book but it has to remain on our do not touch page. Caffeine will slow you down and it will ultimately ruin your game.

It may even keep you from staying hydrated in the long run too.

3. Keep yourself away from foods that you know upset your body. While these foods may seem healthy and helpful to you, they can cause your stomach to hurt, your body to begin to concentrate on healing and loss of performance edge.

This would include any food that gives you gas, things like raw vegetables, beans and popcorn. You know your body and what you should avoid.

4.   Fatty foods. We have talked a great deal about the harmful effects of fatty foods in your diet as an athlete. It has to be on our list here because of the amount of performance success it is likely to steal from you.

This would include foods that are high in saturated fats like creams, fatty meats, deep fried products, and high fat dairy products.

Cut out these products from your diet and you will ultimately have a better result overall for all of your hard work.

Chapter 10: Supplements

Supplements are something that many people wonder about. Are they good for you? Will they enhance my performance? Are they fair to take?

There are many various types of supplements on the market. The goal of any supplement is to supplement your diet. This means it will provide for your diet what you may not already have.

In that, it goes without saying that natural is always going to be better for you. That means that it is a much better option for you to insure that you have a high quality of natural foods in your diet rather than having a bag full of vitamins and minerals that you have to take.

Do I Take Them Or Not?

Only you can truly answer if supplements are in fact right for you and your needs. There is no easy to way to answer this question but we can break it down to help you to understand both points of view.

As an athlete, your body will demand more nutrients including vitamins and minerals of all sorts. It needs this as well as additional calories to keep up with your demand.

It is not simplistic to handle this need though. The best way to get the things you need to balance your diet is to get it from natural, whole foods. To do this, you need to really concentrate on what you need, what is included in what you eat and then insure it is all balanced for optimum nutrition.

That is not an easy task to do, though. Not only do you need to increase the levels of calories that you consume, but you also need to consider the various minerals and vitamins your body needs to make that happen.

Not sure what we mean?

- Niacin

- Iron

- Riboflavin

- Thiamin

That's just to name the most essential.

In most cases, if you can eat a well balanced diet full of vegetables and variety, you can achieve these needs while doing it.

But, if you can not commit to this level of dedication, then providing yourself with a solid supplement can be helpful. Yet, you still have to pay attention to what you are taking.

When purchasing vitamins, you need to make sure that they are the highest of quality and that they are easily absorbed into your body. They should be purchased form a health food store or someplace that is designed for optimum health products.

Beware!

Some vitamins can be dangerous if you take too much of them. This can do the exact opposite of what you are trying to accomplish. If this is something you are not sure about, seeking out the help of a dietician, your pharmacist or even your doctor.

Vitamins are powerful things and they need to be kept regulated for your own safety.

Another reason to speak with your doctor is to insure you are not deficient in any of your vitamins as well. This will help you to balance yourself naturally and therefore find the best success overall.

Conclusion

Sports nutrition is a complex matter. What is important to you and your body is likely not going to be important or as important to someone else.

It can not be stressed enough that the athlete should have a complete health physical done to insure that he is ready to pursue his athletic dreams and his physical height of perfection.

The goal of a physical should be to rule out any conditions that may hinder you but it also should provide information about your needs.

You can learn about your nutritional needs, based on your specific body type and your

ability to meet any deficiency
that you may have.

When it comes to sports
nutrition, there are few things
that are 100% accurate about it.
The fact is that we are all
different people and that means
that our lives and our goals are
all different.

With that too comes the fact that
your body is uniquely yours and
even if you follow a diet
perfectly, it may react differently
to the conditions you present.

Yet, when we condition ourselves
from a nutritional standpoint,
following basic rules of
maintaining healthy bodies, we
will see our bodies improve.

Over time, your body will
become stealthily built to take on

whatever physical challenges
that you provide for it.

Your body will be honed to fit
each of your demands to the
level of perfection you crave.
And, with it will come the highest
level of success you can achieve
both physically and mentally.

Remember, though, that this will
not come without a price to pay.
You will need to work for it and
you will need sheer dedications
to make it happen. In the end,
this is what will define you and
your needs.

Dedication to your sports
nutrition is the foundation of
everything that goes into being
an athlete.

www.ingramcontent.com/pod-product-compliance
Lightning Source LLC
Chambersburg PA
CBHW072147280526
45788CB00002B/800